The Mediterranean Diet for a Better Life

Tasty recipes to enjoy the Mediterranean flavors and have a healthier lifestyle

Lana Green

o

Table of Contents

Kale Salad with Pecorino and Lemon

Prep Time: 5 min

Cook Time: 0 min

Serve: 4

Ingredients:

- 1 large bunch kale, washed and trimmed of steams

- lemons, juiced

- ounces Pecorino Romano, grated

- ½ cup olive oil

- Kosher salt and fresh black pepper to taste

Preparation:

1. Wrap several cabbage leaves lengthwise and cut off the thick central stem using the tip of a knife. On the other hand, wrap the remaining pile of dehydrated leaves in a tight cigar shape and cut them into thin ribbons.

2. Discard the grated cabbage with the cheese. Lightly beat the lemon juice and olive oil and pour over the salad. Try and season with salt and pepper. Let the salad sit at room temperature for an hour before serving.

Venison Tenderloin

Prep Time: 20 min

Cook Time: 75 min

Serve: 6

Ingredients:

- 4 pounds venison tenderloin

- 2 sprigs fresh thyme

- 2 sprigs fresh rosemary

- Two cloves garlic, crushed

- Two bay leaves

- One medium onion, chopped

- 1 cup red wine

- ½ cup apple cider vinegar

Preparation:

1. Add red wine cider vinegar, garlic, bay leaves, thyme, rosemary & onion in a cup & blend them. Move it to the large jar, & place in the bag the venison tenderloin.

2. Close it tightly, and make it airtight. Then place the meat in a refrigerator for marination for at least 13 hours, turn it 2 or 3 times. Preheated the oven to 325°F (165 °C).

3. Take Off meat away from the marinade & put it in a roasting rack. Roast it for two to two and a half hours in the oven. The Internal roasting temperature would be a minimum of 150 °F.

4. Let the roast rest for 10 to 15 minutes before cutting.

5. Heat the sauce over low heat in a pan as the side roasts.

6. Boil till there is a 1/3 drop in the oil. Serve & Enjoy.

Seared venison with plum ginger sauce and vermicelli sauce

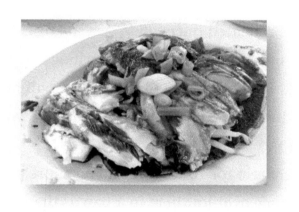

Prep Time: 10 min

Cook Time: 15 min

Serve: 2

Ingredients:

- Vermicelli salad

- One carrot grated

- One red capsicum sliced

- 100 g snow peas sliced

- 100 g vermicelli noodles

- Two tbsp Thai basil leaves chopped

- Venison and plum sauce

- ¼ cup red wine

- One clove garlic minced

- One tablespoon soy sauce

- One teaspoon ginger finely grated

- Two tablespoons plum jam

- 300 g venison medallions

Dressing:

- ½ teaspoon sesame oil

- One tablespoon olive oil

- One tablespoon soy sauce

- One teaspoon plum jam

- One tablespoon Thai basil leaves chopped

- One tablespoon sesame seeds

Preparation:

1. Bring to the boil a full pot.

2. Use a Proof heat Bowl, place the vermicelli noodles in the bowl and pour over the boiling water to cover them. Threads are detached by stirring, covering with a plate, and leaving until smooth, around 4 minutes. Threads are shortened by cutting the threads from different places using kitchen scissors. Apply oil in a small amount to avoid Sticking.

3. Use paper towels, Dry the venison, and season it with salt. 4. Heat the saucepan to medium temperature. Toast sesame seeds until crispy and fragrant for 1 to 2 minutes. Add a drizzle of oil and raise the heat. Once cooked, grill the venison for 2 to 3 minutes on both sides. Cover the venison with foil.

5. Return the pan to low heat for the plum sauce and apply a small amount of oil. Fry the ginger and garlic for 30 seconds, stir-fry the red wine, and boil until halved. Now add plum jelly, fresh plums, and soy sauce and boil until slightly thickened, and stir for around 1 minute. Use black pepper for seasoning. If the sauce gets too thick and jam-like, give a splash of water to thin it out to a decent pouring consistency. Stir in the sleeping venison juices.

6. Mix all of the ingredients in a big dish. Add all the salad ingredients leftover, the noodles, and toss to coat. Season with salt and pepper.

7. Divide the vermicelli salad between the plates to serve. Cover with venison and drizzle all over the sauce with plum.

8. Sprinkle the Thai basil and sesame seeds.

Venison Stir-Fry

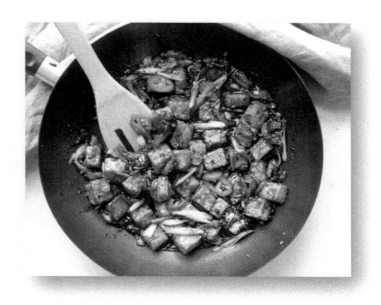

Prep Time: 20 min

Cook Time: 5 min

Serve: 4

Ingredients:

Marinade

- 1/2 teaspoon salt

- Two tablespoons

- Shaoxing wine or dry sherry

- Three tablespoons soy sauce

- One tablespoon potato starch Stir fry

- 1 1/2 cups peanut or other cooking oil

- 1 pound venison, trimmed of fat

- 1 to 4 fresh red chiles

- One red or yellow bell pepper, sliced

- Three garlic cloves, slivered

- One bunch cilantro, roughly chopped

- One tablespoon soy sauce

- Two teaspoons sesame oil

Preparation:

1. Cut the venison into small slivers between 1/4 inch or less and 1 to 3 inches in length from anywhere. Mix and set aside with the marinade as you cut out all the remaining ingredients.

2. Heat a big heavy pot with the peanut oil until it reaches 275 °F to 290°F. Apply about 1/3 of venison to hot oil and use a chopstick or a butter knife to separate the meat slices.

3. Let them sizzle for 30 - 60 seconds. Set aside and cook one-third at a time for the remaining venison.

4. Pour all but only three tablespoons of the oil out of it.

5. Keep the remaining oil hot. Add up the chiles and the bell peppers. Stir-fry for 90 seconds when it starts to burn, add garlic, and cook for an extra 30 seconds. Add the venison and fry for 90 seconds and stir.

6. Add the coriander and soy sauce and fry for the remaining 30 seconds before the coriander wilts. Turn the heat off, then whisk in the sesame oil. Serve with steamed rice at once.

Lamb, apricot & shallot tagine

Prep Time: 30 min

Cook Time: 7 h 30 min

Serve: 5-6

Ingredients:

- 1 tbsp clear honey

- 1 tbsp ras el hanout

- One large leg of lamb, bone-in (about 2kg)

- 150ml hot chicken stock

- Two preserved lemons

- 400g small apricot, halved and stoned

- 600g shallot, halved if particularly large

- 85g whole skinless almond

- couscous and natural yogurt, to serve little pack coriander leaves picked

For the marinade

- 1 tbsp ground cumin

- 2 tbsp clear honey

- 1 tsp coriander seed

- 2 tsp ground cinnamon

- 2 tsp ground ginger

- 4 tbsp olive oil

- Four garlic cloves, crushed pinch of saffron strands

Preparation:

1. Cut the lamb's leg all over and put it in a large bag of food. 2. Using the pestle and mortar, shatter the marinade ingredients simultaneously. Brush over the entire lamb with black pepper. Overnight, or up to 24 hours, to marinate.

3. Place the lamb in a large roasting tin, removing any residual marinade from the top. Use foil to protect the container, and close the foil from the ends. Cook for 6-7 hours, basting until the beef is extremely tender.

4. Drop the oven roasting tin and raise the oven to 200°C /180°C. Pour into a measuring jug the juices from the

lamb, slightly cool it, and remove the fat off. Place the shallots with the lamb in the tin and toss in some of the juices to coat them. Roast the apricots and almonds for 15 mins, and then add them. Whisk the lemon, honey, ras el hanout, and stock in the cooking juices, then pour on the lamb and then roast again for 20 mins.

5. Leave it for 10 minutes, then scatter and eat with couscous and yogurt over the herbs.

Flank Steak, Broccoli and Green Bean Stir-Fry

Prep Time: 15 min

Cook Time: 12 min

Ingredients:

- 3 cups cooked brown rice

- Two tablespoons vegetable oil

- Two tablespoons rice vinegar

- One ¼ pound lean beef flank steak

- 1 cup beef broth

- One tablespoon cornstarch

- One head broccoli, cut into florets (about 6 cups)

- 1 cup shredded carrot

- ½ teaspoon red pepper flakes

- ½ teaspoon Chinese five-spice powder

- ½ pound thin green beans, trimmed

- ½ large onion, sliced

- ½ cup sliced almonds

- ¼ teaspoon salt

- ¼ cup reduced-sodium soy sauce

Preparation:

1. Combine the soy sauce, broth, 5-spice powder, vinegar, cornstarch, & the red chili flakes in a cup and place it aside.

2. Take a non-stick fry pan, add 1 tbsp of oil to it, and heat it. Pepper the salted stir-fry flank steak & for 4 minutes. Remove to a tray. Add the remaining one tbsp. Of oil in it, and then add broccoli, cabbage, green beans, & carrot. Stir-cook for 9 minutes or till it becomes soft & crisp.

3. Add ¼ cup of water at the last two minutes of cooking time. Now add a mixture of soya sauce& broth in it and then boil & simmer it for 2 minutes, until well dense. Stir in some stored juices & beef & heat up. Decorate with the almonds & serve with the cooked brown rice instantly.

Moroccan beef tagine

Prep Time: 25 min

Cook Time: 7 hrs

Serve: 4

Ingredients:

Marinade

- pinch of sea salt
- pinch of ground cardamon
- 1 tsp ground sweet paprika
- 1 tsp ground ginger
- 1 tsp ground cumin
- 1 tsp ground cinnamon
- 1 tsp dried rose petals
- 1 tbsp ras el hanout
- 1 tbsp olive oil

Tagine

- One onion, peeled and chopped
- 1 tbsp olive oil for frying
- 400 g of chickpeas
- 400 g chopped tomatoes
- 150 g prunes, sliced
- 150 ml of beef stock
- Two carrots sliced
- Four small tomatoes quartered
- 400 g butternut squash, diced
- 600 g diced stewing beef
- fresh coriander

Preparation:

1. Combine all marinade items in a small glass.

2. Take a dish, place beef in it, pour marinade all over it & mix it well for coating all-beef parts equally.

3. Cover bowl with foil & refrigerate it for 3 to 4 hours.

4. Take a frying pan, add oil in it, heat it, add onions and fry for 3 to 4 minutes, then add beef in it and fry it for 5 to 6 minutes until it turned brown.

5. In a boiled slow oven dish, pass by the onion & beef.

6. Add & stock the tinned tomatoes along with onions, quartered tomatoes &, stir well, add the onions, quartered tomatoes, & butternut squash, & then mix again.

7. Turn on the auto mode, cover a slow cooker, & keep a dish simmer for 7 to 8 hours until the beef is very tender. Add the prunes & chickpeas for one hour till cooking ends. Serve with splattered couscous with finely sliced coriander.

Persian Roast Lamb

Prep Time: 20 min

Cook Time: 150 min

Serve: 8

Ingredients:

- One large onion sliced or chopped

- 1 tbsp EV olive oil

- 1 tbsp ground cumin

- tsp ground black pepper

- 1 tsp turmeric

- One leg or shoulder of lamb

- Two strips of fresh rosemary

- 2 Tbsp honey

- Tbsp liquid saffron

- 250 ml of vegetable stock

- 4 tbsp pomegranate molasses

- Five cloves garlic finely chopped or crushed

- One lemon juice

- Marinade

Preparation:

1. Preheat micro to 180 deg C. Make slashes. Mix ingredients & rub them over the lamb.

2. Line sliced onions with a preferred dish. Pour the stock.

3. Remember to Pour on onions. Cover using foil & roast for 60 minutes. Have the lamb wrapped in aluminum foil with a wonderful sauce.

Stir-fried garlic chili beef and ong Choi

Prep Time: 8 min

Cook Time: 15 min

Serve: 2

Ingredients:

- 200g beef fillet, sliced into even-sized thin strips

- Few pinches Chinese five-spice

- Light soy sauce to season

- 1 tbsp groundnut oil

- Four large garlic cloves, finely chopped

- 150 ong Choi, washed, leaves and stems cut across the stem in equal 10cm lengths (or use spinach or watercress)

- One medium red chili, de-seeded and finely chopped Toasted sesame oil, to season

Preparation:

1. Season the beef with soy sauce. Toss well. Heat a saucepan. Add oil & garlic. Fry 30 sec. Add beef & stir.

2. Apply one Choi & chili. Season with light soy sauce, sea salt, & sesame oil splashes for serving.

3. Serve immediately & enjoy.

Asian Broccoli and Ginger Salad

Prep Time: 10 min

Cook Time: 10 min

Serve: 4

Ingredients:

- Salt and pepper to taste
- Three tablespoons low sodium soy sauce
- Three tablespoons balsamic vinegar
- Two cloves garlic minced
- Two teaspoons brown sugar
- 2 cups sugar snap peas
- 1/4 cup almonds
- One red pepper julienne cut
- 1 (12 ounces) bag broccoli coleslaw

- One tablespoon fresh ginger

- 1 1/2 teaspoons sesame oil

Preparation:

1. Mix soy sauce, garlic, sesame oil, vinegar, brown sugar, & ginger. Put it aside for a while. Steam sugar snaps for roughly 3-4 min.

2. For stopping the cooking process, immerse it in an ice bath. Drain well. Mix peas, almonds, broccoli coleslaw, red pepper & sesame ginger. Dressing in a big dish.

3. Add salt to taste & black pepper powder.

Avocado and three-bean salad

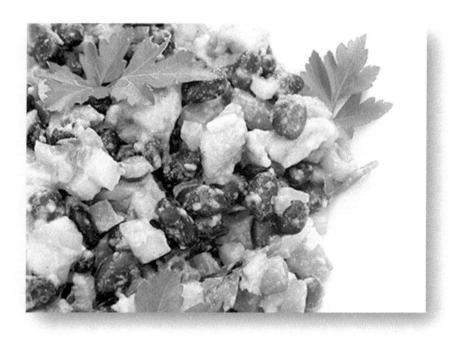

Prep Time: 15 min

Cook Time: 15 min

Serve: 8

Ingredients:

- salt and pepper to taste

- juice of 2 limes

- Two large avocados, peeled, pitted, and diced

- Two cloves garlic, mashed or finely diced

- 12 grape or cherry tomatoes, halved

- 1/3 cup olive oil

- One large orange or red bell pepper, diced

- One bunch cilantro, chopped

- 15 oz kernel corn

- 15 oz red kidney beans

- 15 oz garbanzo beans

- 15 oz black beans

Preparation:
1. Take a big bowl. Combine all ingredients. Refrigerate for 60 minutes before serving.
2. Tossed it with lime. Serve & enjoy.

Baked Adzuki Beans with Aubergine & Tomatoes

Prep time: 8 min

Cook time: 90 min

Serve: 6

Ingredients:

- One bouquet garni (thyme, parsley, and bay leaf)

- cup chicken stock (or one bouillon cube dissolved in 1 cup water)

- 1 cup dried adzuki beans

- One onion, finely chopped

- 1⁄2 cup fresh grated parmesan cheese

- 1⁄2 teaspoon ground allspice

- 1⁄4 teaspoon red pepper flakes

- Two cloves garlic, minced

- Two sliced eggplants

- ½ cups canned chopped tomatoes

- Four tablespoons fresh basil, shredded

- Six tablespoons olive oil

- kosher salt or sea salt

- salt and pepper, to taste

Preparation:

1. Add garlic & boil water. Reduce heat & simmer before beans become soft for 50 minutes. Preheat microwave to 375°. Heat olive oil in a frying pan on moderate heat.

2. Move to bake dish. Heat leftover olive oil pan & sauté onion before it begins to soften.

3. Add garlic & sauté for one min. Add tomatoes, red pepper flakes, salt, allspice, & black pepper. Blend well.

4. Sprinkle with cheese & bake for 20 min. Serve & enjoy.

Roasted Sorghum

Prep Time: 10 min

Cook Time: 15 min

Serve: 4

Ingredients:

- tbsp. avocado oil
- ½ cup sorghum, cooked
- 1 carrot, diced
- tbsp. dried parsley
- ½ tsp. dried oregano
- 2 tbsp. cream cheese

Preparation:

1. Heat avocado oil and add the carrot. Roast it for 5 minutes. Then add cooked sorghum, parsley, oregano, and cream cheese.

2. Roast the meal for 10 minutes on low heat. Stir it from time to time to avoid burning.

Sorghum Stew

Prep Time: 10 min

Cook Time: 25 min

Serve: 5

Ingredients:

- 1 cup sorghum
- ½ cup ground sausages
- ½ cup tomatoes
- 1 jalapeno pepper, chopped
- ½ cup bell pepper, chopped
- 4 cups chicken stock

Preparation:

1. Roast the sausages for 5 minutes in the saucepan. Then add tomatoes, jalapeno, and bell pepper.

Cook the ingredients for 10 minutes.

2. After this, add sorghum and chicken stock and boil the stew for 10 minutes more.

Sorghum Salad

Prep Time: 10 min

Cook Time: 10 min

Serve: 3

Ingredients:

- 3 oz butternut squash, chopped

- ¼ cup sorghum

- ¼ cup fresh cilantro, chopped

- 1 tsp. ground cumin

- cups water

- 2 tbsp. organic canola oil

- 2 tbsp. apple cider vinegar

Preparation:

1. Put sorghum and butternut squash in the saucepan. Add water and cook for 10 minutes. Then cool the ingredients and transfer in the salad bowl.

2. Add cilantro, ground cumin, organic canola oil, and apple cider vinegar. Stir the meal well.

Sorghum Bake

Prep Time: 10 min

Cook Time: 25 min

Serve: 4

Ingredients:

- ½ cup sorghum

- 1 apple, chopped

- 1 oz raisins

- 1.5cup of water

Preparation:

1. Put sorghum in the pan. Flatten it. Then top it with raisins, apple, and water. Cover the meal with baking paper and transfer in the preheated to 375F oven.

2. Bake the meal for 25 minutes.

Lamb and Chickpeas Stew

Prep Time: 10 min

Cook Time: 1 h 20 min

Serve: 6

Ingredients:

- 1 and ½ lb. lamb shoulder, cubed

- 3 tbsp. olive oil

- 1 cup yellow onion, chopped

- 1 cup carrots, cubed

- 1 cup celery, chopped

- 3 garlic cloves, minced

- 4 rosemary springs, chopped

- 2 cups chicken stock

- 1 cup tomato puree

- 15 oz. canned chickpeas, drained and rinsed

- 10 oz. baby spinach

- 2 tbsp. black olives, pitted and sliced

- A pinch of salt and black pepper

Preparation:

1. Heat a pot with the oil over medium-high heat, add the meat, salt and pepper and brown for 5 minutes.

2. Add carrots, celery, onion and garlic, stir and sauté for 5 minutes more. Add the rosemary, stock, chickpeas and the other ingredients except the spinach and olives, stir and cook for 1 hour.

3. Add the rest of the ingredients, cook the stew over medium heat for 10 minutes more, divide into bowls and serve.

Chorizo and Lentils Stew

Prep Time: 10 min

Cook Time: 35 min

Serve: 4

Ingredients:

- 4 cups water

- 1 cup carrots, sliced

- 1 yellow onion, chopped

- 1 tbsp. extra-virgin olive oil

- ¾ cup celery, chopped

- 1 and ½ tsp. garlic, minced

- 1 and ½ lb. gold potatoes, roughly chopped

- 7 oz. chorizo, cut in half lengthwise and thinly sliced

- 1 and ½ cup lentils

- ½ tsp. smoked paprika

- ½ tsp. oregano

- Salt and black pepper to taste

- 14 oz. canned tomatoes, chopped

- ½ cup cilantro, chopped

Preparation:

1. Heat a saucepan with oil over medium high heat, add onion, garlic, celery and carrots, stir and cook for 4 minutes.

2. Add the chorizo, stir and cook for 1 minute more.

3. Add the rest of the ingredients except the cilantro, stir, bring to a boil, reduce heat to medium-low and simmer for 25 minutes. Divide the stew into bowls and serve with the cilantro sprinkled on top. Enjoy!

Lamb and Potato Stew

Prep Time: 10 min

Cook Time: 2 h

Serve: 4

Ingredients:

- 2 and ½ lb. lamb shoulder, boneless and cut in small pieces Salt and black pepper to taste
- 1 yellow onion, chopped
- 3 tbsp. extra virgin olive oil
- 3 tomatoes, grated
- and ½ cups chicken stock
- ½ cup dry white wine
- 1 bay leaf
- ½ lb. gold potatoes, cut into medium cubes
- ¾ cup green olives

Preparation:

1. Heat a saucepan with the oil over medium high heat, add the lamb, brown for 10 minutes, transfer to a platter and keep warm for now. Heat the pan again, add onion, stir and cook for 4 minutes. Add tomatoes, stir, reduce heat to low and cook for 15 minutes.

2. Return lamb meat to pan, add wine and the rest of the ingredients except the potatoes and olives, stir, increase heat to medium high, bring to a boil, reduce heat again, cover pan and simmer for 30 minutes.

3. Add potatoes and olives, stir, cook for 1 more hour, divide into bowls and serve.

Meatball and Pasta Soup

Prep Time: 10 min

Cook Time: 40 min

Serve: 4

Ingredients:

- 12 oz. pork meat, ground

- 12 oz. veal, ground

- Salt and black pepper to taste

- 1 garlic clove, minced

- garlic cloves, sliced

- 2 tsp. thyme, chopped

- 1 egg, whisked

- oz. Manchego, grated

- 2 tbsp. extra virgin olive oil

- 1/3 cup panko

- 4 cups chicken stock

- A pinch of saffron

- 15 oz. canned tomatoes, crushed

- 1 tbsp. parsley, chopped

- 8 oz. pasta

Preparation:

1. In a bowl, mix veal with pork, 1 garlic clove, 1 tsp. thyme, ¼ tsp. paprika, salt, pepper to taste, egg, manchego, panko, stir very well and shape medium meatballs out of this mix.

2. Heat a pan with 1 ½ tbsp. oil over medium high heat, add half of the meatballs, cook for 2 minutes on each side, transfer to paper towels, drain grease and put on a plate.

3. Repeat this with the rest of the meatballs.

4. Heat a saucepan with the rest of the oil, add sliced garlic, stir and cook for 1 minute.

5. Add the remaining ingredients and the meatballs, stir, reduce heat to medium low, cook for 25 minutes and season with salt and pepper. Cook pasta according to instructions, drain, put in a bowl and mix with ½ cup soup.

6. Divide pasta into soup bowls, add soup and meatballs on top, sprinkle parsley all over and serve.

Peas Soup

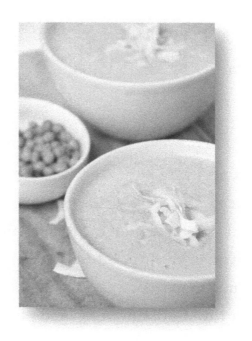

Prep Time: 10 min

Cook Time: 10 min

Serve: 4

Ingredients:

- 1 tsp. shallot, chopped

- 1 tbsp. butter

- quart chicken stock

- 2 eggs

- 3 tbsp. lemon juice

- 2 cups peas

- tbsp. parmesan, grated

- Salt and black pepper to taste

Preparation:

1. Heat a saucepan with the butter over medium high heat, add shallot, stir and cook for 2 minutes.
2. Add stock, lemon juice, some salt and pepper and the whisked eggs.
3. Add more salt and pepper to taste, peas and parmesan cheese, stir, cook for 3 minutes, divide into bowls and serve.

Minty Lamb Stew

Prep Time: 10 min

Cook Time: 1 h 45 min

Serve: 4

Ingredients:

- cups orange juice

- ½ cup mint tea

- Salt and black pepper to taste

- 2 lb. lamb shoulder chops

- 1 tbsp. mustard, dry

- 3 tbsp. canola oil

- 1 tbsp. ras el hanout

- 1 carrot, chopped

- 1 yellow onion, chopped

- 1 celery rib, chopped

- 1 tbsp. ginger, grated

- 28 oz. canned tomatoes, crushed

- 1 tbsp. garlic, minced

- star anise

- 1 cup apricots, dried and cut in halves

- 1 cinnamon stick

- ½ cup mint, chopped

- 15 oz. canned chickpeas, drained

- 6 tbsp. yogurt

Preparation:

1. Put orange juice in a saucepan, bring to a boil over medium heat, take off heat, add tea leaves, cover and leave aside for 3 minutes, strain this and leave aside.

2. Heat a saucepan with 2 tbsp. oil over medium high heat, add lamb chops seasoned with salt, pepper, mustard and rasel hanout, toss, brown for 3 minutes on each side and transfer to a plate. Add remaining oil to the saucepan, heat over medium heat, add ginger, onion, carrot, garlic and celery, stir and cook for 5 minutes.

3. Add orange juice, star anise, tomatoes, cinnamon stick, lamb, apricots, stir and cook for 1 hour and 30 minutes.

4. Transfer lamb chops to a cutting board, discard bones and chop. Bring sauce from the pan to a boil, add chickpeas and mint, stir and cook for 10 minutes.

5. Discard cinnamon and star anise, divide into bowls and serve with yogurt on top.

Spinach and Orzo Soup

Prep Time: 10 min

Cook Time: 10 min

Serve: 4

Ingredients:

- ½ cup orzo

- 6 cups chicken soup

- and ½ cups parmesan, grated

- Salt and black pepper to taste

- 1 and ½ tsp. oregano, dried

- ¼ cup yellow onion, finely chopped

- 3 cups baby spinach

- tbsp. lemon juice

- ½ cup peas, frozen

Preparation:

1. Heat a saucepan with the stock over high heat, add oregano, orzo, onion, salt and pepper, stir, bring to a boil, cover and cook for 10 minutes.

2. Take soup off the heat, add salt and pepper to taste and the rest of the ingredients, stir well and divide into soup bowls. Serve right away.

Minty Lentil and Spinach Soup

Prep Time: 10 min

Cook Time: 30 min

Serve: 6

Ingredients:

- 2 tbsp. olive oil
- 1 yellow onion, chopped
- A pinch of salt and black pepper
- 2 garlic cloves, minced
- 1 tsp. coriander, ground
- 1 tsp. cumin, ground
- 1 tsp. sumac
- 1 tsp. red pepper, crushed
- 2 tsp. mint, dried
- 1 tbsp. flour
- 6 cups veggie stock

- 3 cups water

- 12 oz. spinach, torn

- 1 and ½ cups brown lentils, rinsed

- 2 cups parsley, chopped

- Juice of 1 lime

Preparation:

1. Heat a pot with the oil over medium heat, add the onions, stir and sauté for 5 minutes.

2. Add garlic, salt, pepper, coriander, cumin, sumac, red pepper, mint and flour, stir and cook for another minute.

3.. Add the stock, water and the other ingredients except the parsley and lime juice, stir, bring to a simmer and cook for 20 minutes. Add the parsley and lime juice, cook the soup for 5 minutes more, ladle into bowls and serve.

Chicken and Apricots Stew

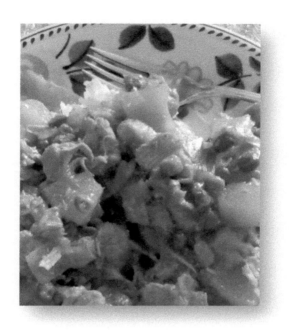

Prep Time: 10 min

Cook Time: 2 h 10 min

Serve: 4

Ingredients:

- 3 garlic cloves, minced

- 1 tbsp. parsley, chopped

- 20 saffron threads

- 3 tbsp. cilantro, chopped

- Salt and black pepper to taste

- 1 tsp. ginger, ground

- tbsp. olive oil

- red onions, thinly sliced

- 4 chicken drumsticks

- 5 oz. apricots, dried

- 2 tbsp. butter

- ¼ cup honey

- 2/3 cup walnuts, chopped

- ½ cinnamon stick

Preparation:

1. Heat a pan over medium high heat, add saffron threads, toast them for 2 minutes, transfer to a bowl, cool down and crush. Add the chicken pieces, 1 tbsp. cilantro, parsley, garlic, ginger, salt, pepper, oil and 2 tbsp. water, toss well and keep in the fridge for 30 minutes.

2. Arrange onion on the bottom of a saucepan.

3. Add chicken and marinade, add 1 tbsp. butter, place on stove over medium high heat and cook for 15 minutes.

4. Add ¼ cup water, stir, cover pan, reduce heat to medium- low and simmer for 45 minutes.

5. Heat a pan over medium heat, add 2 tbsp. honey, cinnamon stick, apricots and ¾ cup water, stir, bring to a boil, reduce to low and simmer for 15 minutes.

6. Take off heat, discard cinnamon and leave to cool down.

7. Heat a pan with remaining butter over medium heat, add remaining honey and walnuts, stir, cook for 5 minutes and transfer to a plate. Add chicken to apricot sauce, also season with salt, pepper and the rest of the cilantro stir, cook for 10 minutes and serve on top of walnuts.

Fish and Veggie Stew

Prep Time: 10 min

Cook Time: 1 h 30 min

Serve: 4

Ingredients:

- 6 lemon wedges, pulp separated and chopped and some of the peel reserved
- 2 tbsp. parsley, chopped
- 2 tomatoes, cut in halves, peeled and grated
- 2 tbsp. cilantro, chopped
- 2 garlic cloves, minced
- ½ tsp. paprika
- 2 tbsp. water
- ½ cup water
- ½ tsp. cumin, ground
- Salt and black pepper to taste

- 4 bass fillets

- ¼ cup olive oil

- 3 carrots, sliced

- 1 red bell pepper, sliced lengthwise and thinly cut in strips

- 1 and ¼ lb. potatoes, peeled and sliced

- ½ cup olives

- 1 red onion, thinly sliced

Preparation:

1. In a bowl, mix tomatoes with lemon pulp, cilantro, parsley, cumin, garlic, paprika, salt, pepper, 2 tbsp. water, 2 tsp. oil and the fish, toss to coat and keep in the fridge for 30 minutes. Heat a saucepan with the water and some salt over medium high heat, add potatoes and carrots, stir, cook for 10 minutes and drain.

2. Heat a pan over medium heat, add bell pepper and ¼ cup water, cover, cook for 5 minutes and take off heat.

3. Coat a saucepan with remaining oil, add potatoes and carrots, ¼ cup water, onion slices, fish and its marinade,

bell pepper strips, olives, salt and pepper, toss gently, cook for 45 minutes, divide into bowls and serve.

Tomato Soup

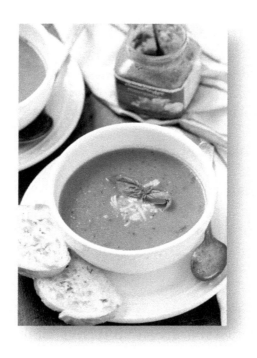

Prep Time: 60 min

Cook Time: 2 min

Serve: 4

Ingredients:

- ½ green bell pepper, chopped

- ½ red bell pepper, chopped

- 1 and ¾ lb. tomatoes, chopped

- ¼ cup bread, torn

- 9 tbsp. extra virgin olive oil

- 1 garlic clove, minced

- 2 tsp. sherry vinegar

- Salt and black pepper to taste

- 1 tbsp. cilantro, chopped

- A pinch of cumin, ground

Preparation:

1. In a blender, mix green and red bell peppers with tomatoes, salt, pepper, 6 tbsp. oil, and the other ingredients except the bread and cilantro, and pulse well. Keep in the fridge for 1 hour.

2. Heat a pan with remaining oil over medium high heat, add bread pieces, and toast them for 1 minute.

3. Divide cold soup into bowls, top with bread cubes and cilantro then serve.

Chickpeas Soup

Prep Time: 10 min

Cook Time: 35 min

Serve: 4

Ingredients:

- 1 bunch kale, leaves torn
- Salt and black pepper to taste
- 3 tbsp. olive oil
- 1 celery stalk, chopped
- 1 yellow onion, chopped
- 1 carrot, chopped
- 30 oz. canned chickpeas, drained
- 14 oz. canned tomatoes, chopped
- 1 bay leaf
- 3 rosemary sprigs
- 4 cups veggie stock

Preparation:

1. In a bowl, mix kale with half of the oil, salt and pepper, toss to coat., spread on a lined baking sheet, cook at 425°F for 12 minutes and leave aside to cool down.

2. Heat a saucepan with remaining oil over medium high heat, add carrot, celery, onion, salt and pepper, and stir and cook for 5 minutes. Add the rest of the ingredients, toss and simmer for 20 minutes.

3. Discard rosemary and bay leaf, puree using a blender and divide into soup bowls. Top with roasted kale and serve.

Fish Soup

Prep Time: 10 min

Cook Time: 35 min

Serve: 6

Ingredients:

- 2 garlic cloves, minced

- 2 tbsp. olive oil

- 1 fennel bulb, sliced

- 1 yellow onion, chopped

- 1 pinch saffron, soaked in some orange juice for 10 minutes and drained

- 14 oz. canned tomatoes, peeled

- 1 strip orange zest

- 6 cups seafood stock

- 10 halibut fillet, cut into big pieces

- 20 shrimp, peeled and deveined

- 1 bunch parsley, chopped

- Salt and white pepper to taste

Preparation:

1. 2. Heat a saucepan with oil over medium high heat, add onion, garlic and fennel, stir and cook for 10 minutes.

Add saffron, tomatoes, orange zest and stock, stir, bring to a boil and simmer for 20 minutes.

3. Add fish and shrimp, stir and cook for 6 minutes.

4. Sprinkle parsley, salt and pepper, divide into bowls and serve.

Chili Watermelon Soup

Prep Time: 4 h

Cook Time: 5 min

Serve: 4

Ingredients:

- 3 lb. watermelon, sliced
- ½ tsp. chipotle chili powder
- 2 tbsp. olive oil
- Salt to taste
- 1 tomato, chopped
- 1 tbsp. shallot, chopped
- ¼ cup cilantro, chopped
- 1 small cucumber, chopped
- 1 small Serrano chili pepper, chopped
- 3 and ½ tbsp. lime juice

- ¼ cup crème Fraiche

- ½ tbsp. red wine vinegar

Preparation:

1. In a bowl, mix 1 tbsp. oil with chipotle powder, stir and brush the watermelon with this mix. Put the watermelon slices preheated grill pan over medium high heat, grill for 1 minute on each side, cool down, chop and put in a blender.

2. Add cucumber and the rest of the ingredients except the vinegar and the lime juice and pulse well.

3. Transfer to bowls, top with lime juice and vinegar, keep in the fridge for 4 hours and then serve.

Shrimp Soup

Prep Time: 30 min

Cook Time: 5 min

Serve: 6

Ingredients:

- 1 English cucumber, chopped

- 3 cups tomato juice

- 3 jarred roasted red peppers, chopped

- ½ cup olive oil

- 2 tbsp. sherry vinegar

- 1 tsp. sherry vinegar

- garlic clove, mashed

- baguette slices, cut into cubes and toasted

- Salt and black pepper to taste

- ½ tsp. cumin, ground

- ¾ lb. shrimp, peeled and deveined

- 1 tsp. thyme, chopped

Preparation:

1. In a blender, mix cucumber with tomato juice, red peppers and pulse well, bread, 6 tbsp. oil, 2 tbsp. vinegar, cumin, salt, pepper and garlic, pulse again, transfer to a bowl and keep in the fridge for 30 minutes.

2. Heat a saucepan with 1 tbsp. oil over high heat, add shrimp, stir and cook for 2 minutes. Add thyme, and the rest of the ingredients, cook for 1 minute and transfer to a plate.

3. Divide cold soup into bowls, top with shrimp and serve.

Halibut and Veggies Stew

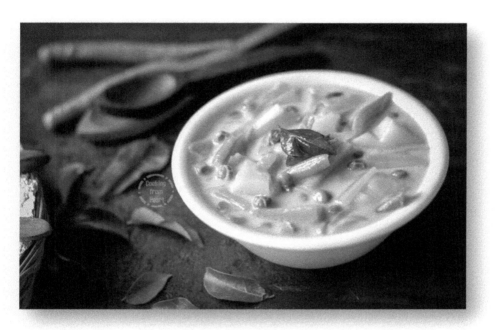

Prep Time: 10 min

Cook Time: 50 min

Serve: 4

Ingredients:

- 1 yellow onion, chopped

- 2 tbsp. oil

- 1 fennel bulb, stalks removed, sliced and roughly chopped
- 1 carrot, thinly sliced crosswise
- 1 red bell pepper, chopped
- 2 garlic cloves, minced
- 3 tbsp. tomato paste
- 16 oz. canned chickpeas, drained
- ½ cup dry white wine
- tsp. thyme, chopped
- A pinch of smoked paprika
- Salt and black pepper to taste
- 1 bay leaf
- pinches saffron
- 4 baguette slices, toasted
- 3 and ½ cups water
- 13 mussels, debearded
- 11 oz. halibut fillets, skinless and cut into chunks

Preparation:

1. Heat a saucepan with the oil over medium high heat, add fennel, onion, bell pepper, garlic, tomato paste and carrot, stir and cook for 5 minutes.

2. Add wine, stir and cook for 2 minutes. Add the rest of the ingredients except the halibut and mussels, stir, bring to a boil, cover and boil for 25 minutes. Add, halibut and mussels, cover and simmer for 6 minutes more.

3. Discard unopened mussels, ladle into bowls and serve with toasted bread on the side.

Cucumber Soup

Prep Time: 10 min

Cook Time: 6 min

Serve: 4

Ingredients:

- 3 bread slices

- ¼ cup almonds

- 4 tsp. almonds

- 3 cucumbers, peeled and chopped

- 3 garlic cloves, minced

- ½ cup warm water

- 6 scallions, thinly sliced

- ¼ cup white wine vinegar

- 3 tbsp. olive oil

- Salt to taste

- 1 tsp. lemon juice

- ½ cup green grapes, cut in halves

Preparation:

1. Heat a pan over medium high heat, add almonds, stir, toast for 5 minutes, transfer to a plate and leave aside.

2. Soak bread in warm water for 2 minutes, transfer to a blender, add almost all the cucumber, salt, the oil, garlic, 5 scallions, lemon juice, vinegar and half of the almonds and pulse well. Ladle soup into bowls, top with reserved ingredients and 2 tbsp. grapes and serve.

Chickpeas, Tomato and Kale Stew

Prep Time: 10 min

Cook Time: 30 min

Serve: 4

Ingredients:

- 1 yellow onion, chopped

- tbsp. extra-virgin olive oil

- cups sweet potatoes, peeled and chopped

- 1 ½ tsp. cumin, ground

- 4-inch cinnamon stick

- 14 oz. canned tomatoes, chopped

- 14 oz. canned chickpeas, drained 1 ½ tsp. honey

- 6 tbsp. orange juice 1 cup water

- Salt and black pepper to taste

- ½ cup green olives, pitted

- 2 cups kale leaves, chopped

Preparation:

1. Heat a saucepan with the oil over medium high heat, add onion, cumin and cinnamon stir and cook for 5 minutes.

2. Add potatoes and the rest of the ingredients except the kale, stir, cover, reduce heat to medium-low and cook for 15 minutes. Add kale, stir, cover again and cook for 10 minutes more. Divide into bowls and serve.

Veggie Stew

Prep Time: 10 min

Cook Time: 50 min

Serve: 4

Ingredients:

- eggplants, chopped

- Salt and black pepper to taste

- 6 zucchinis, chopped

- 2 yellow onions, chopped

- 3 red bell peppers, chopped

- 56 oz. canned tomatoes, chopped

- A handful black olives, pitted and chopped

- A pinch of allspice, ground

- A pinch of cinnamon, ground

- 1 tsp. oregano, dried

- A drizzle of honey

- 1 tbsp. garbanzo bean flour mixed with

- 1 tbsp. water A drizzle of olive oil

- A pinch of red chili flakes

- 3 tbsp. Greek yogurt

Preparation:

1. Heat a saucepan with the oil over medium high heat, add bell peppers, onions, salt and pepper, and stir and sauté for 4 minutes.

2. Add eggplant and the rest of the ingredients except the flour, olives, chili flakes and the yogurt, stir, bring to a boil, cover, reduce heat to medium-low and cook for 45 minutes.

3. Add the remaining ingredients except the yogurt, stir, cook for 1 minute, divide into bowls and serve with some Greek yogurt on top.

Beef and Eggplant Soup

Prep Time: 10 min

Cook Time: 30 min

Serve: 8

Ingredients:

- 1 yellow onion, chopped

- 1 tbsp. olive oil

- 1 garlic clove, minced

- 1 lb. beef, ground

- 1 lb. eggplant, chopped

- ¾ cup celery, chopped

- ¾ cup carrots, chopped

- Salt and black pepper to taste

- 29 oz. canned tomatoes, drained and chopped

- 28 oz. beef stock

- ½ tsp. nutmeg, ground

- ½ cup macaroni

- 2 tsp. parsley, chopped

- ½ cup parmesan cheese, grated

Preparation:

1. Heat a large saucepan with the oil over medium heat, add onion, garlic and meat, stir and brown for 5 minutes.

2. Add celery, carrots and the other ingredients except the macaroni and the cheese, stir, bring to a simmer and cook for 20 minutes. Add macaroni, stir and cook for 12 minutes.

3. Ladle into soup bowls, top with grated cheese and serve.

Mediterranean Greens Preparation

Prep Time: 10 min

Cook Time: 0 min

Serve: 4

Ingredients:

- 6 cups assorted fresh mixed greens (such as radicchio, arugula, watercress, baby spinach, and romaine)
- 1 small red onion, thinly sliced
- 20 cherry tomatoes, halved
- ¼ cup dried cranberries
- ¼ cup chopped walnuts
- Crumbled feta cheese
- Freshly ground pepper to taste
- 2 tbsp. balsamic vinegar

- 2 cloves fresh garlic, finely minced

- 4 tbsp. extra-virgin olive oil

- 1 tbsp. water

- ½ tsp. crushed dried oregano

Preparation:

1. Take out a large salad bowl, combine walnuts, greens, tomatoes, onion, and cranberries. Gently toss.

2. For the dressing, combine water, vinegar, oregano, olive oil, and garlic. Mix the ingredients well. Pour over the salad and lightly toss. Add feta cheese as garnish, if preferred.

3. Add pepper to taste.

Classic Greek Salad

Prep Time: 15 min

Cook Time: 0 min

Serve: 6

Ingredients:

- 6 large firm tomatoes, quartered

- 20 Greek black olives

- ½ lb. Greek feta cheese, cut into small cubes

- ½ head of escarole, shredded

- 3 tbsp. red wine vinegar

- ¼ cup extra-virgin olive oil

- 1 tbsp. dried oregano

- ½ English cucumber, peeled, seeded, and thinly sliced

- 2 cloves fresh garlic, finely minced

- ½ red onion, sliced

- 1 medium red bell pepper, seeded and sliced

- ¼ cup freshly chopped Italian parsley

- Salt and freshly ground pepper to taste

Preparation:

1. Take out a large bowl and add vinegar, oregano, olive oil, and garlic. Add salt and pepper to taste. Set aside the bowl.

2. In another large bowl, add onion, tomatoes, escarole, cucumber, bell pepper, and cheese and mix them well.

3. Take the vinegar mixture and pour it over the salad in the second bowl. Top the salad with olives and parsley.

North African Zucchini Salad

Prep Time: 10 min

Cook Time: 0 min

Serve: 4

Ingredients:

- 1 lb. firm green zucchini, thinly sliced

- ½ tsp. ground cumin

- 2 cloves fresh garlic, finely minced

- Juice from 1 large lemon

- 1 tbsp. extra-virgin olive oil

- 1½ tbsp. plain low-fat yogurt

- Crumbled feta cheese

- Finely chopped parsley for garnish

- Salt and freshly ground pepper to taste

Preparation:

1. Add the zucchini into a large saucepan and steam it for about 2-5 minutes, or until it becomes tender and crispy. Place the zucchini under cold water and drain well.

2. Take out a large bowl and mix cumin, olive oil, lemon juice, garlic, and yogurt. Add salt and pepper to taste. Add the zucchini into the mixture in the bowl and toss gently.

3. Serve with feta cheese and parsley as garnish.

Tunisian Style Carrot Salad

Prep Time: 15 min

Cook Time: 0 min

Serve: 6

Ingredients:

- 10 medium carrots, peeled and sliced

- 1 cup crumbled feta cheese, divided

- 2 tsp. caraway seed

- ¼ cup extra-virgin olive oil

- 6 tbsp. apple cider vinegar

- 5 tsp. freshly minced garlic

- 1 tbsp. Harissa paste (choose the level of heat based on your preference)

- 20 pitted Kalamata olives, reserving some for garnish

- Salt to taste

Preparation:

1. Take out a medium saucepan and place it on medium heat. Fill it with water and add the carrots. Cook carrots until tender. Drain and cool the carrots under cold water. Drain again to remove any excess water.

2. Take out a large bowl and place the carrots in them.

3. Take out a mortar and combine salt, garlic, and caraway seeds. Grind them until they form a paste. Otherwise, you can also use a small bowl, preferably one not made out of glass for grind. The final option would be to toss the ingredients into a blender and pulse them. Add vinegar and Harissa into the bowl with the carrots and mix them well.

4. Use a large spoon and mash the carrots. Add the garlic mixture into the carrot and mix again until they have all blended well. Add the olive oil and mix again.

5. Finally, add about ½ the feta cheese and all the olives and mix well again. Take out a large bowl and add the salad to it. Top it with the remaining feta cheese.

Caesar Salad

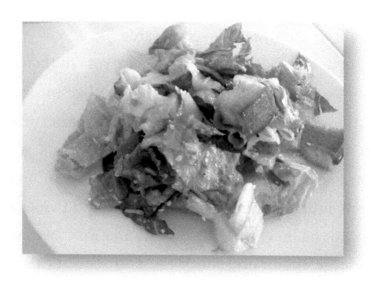

Prep Time: 5 min

Cook Time: 0 min

Serve: 6

Ingredients:

- 10 small pitted black olives, chopped

- 1-2 bunches romaine lettuce, cleaned and torn in pieces

- 2 tsp. lemon juice

- 2½ tsp. balsamic vinegar

- ½ cup grated parmesan cheese

- ½ cup nonfat plain yogurt

- 1 tsp. worcestershire sauce

- ½ tsp. anchovy paste

- 2 cloves freshly minced garlic

Preparation:

1. Take out a large bowl and place romaine lettuce in it.

2. Take out your blended and add mix lemon juice, yogurt, garlic, anchovy paste, vinegar, worcestershire sauce, and ¼ cup parmesan cheese. Mix all the ingredients well until they are smooth.

3. Pour the yogurt mixture over the lettuce and toss lightly.

4. Top the salad with the remaining parmesan cheese.

Cress and Tangerine Salad

Prep Time: 15 min

Cook Time: 0 min

Serve: 4

Ingredients:

- 4 large sweet tangerines

- ¼ cup extra-virgin olive oil

- 2 large bunches watercress, washed and stems removed Juice from 1 fresh lemon

- 10 cherry tomatoes, halved

- 16 pitted Kalamata olives

- Sea salt and freshly ground pepper to taste

Preparation:

1. Take the tangerines and peel them into a medium-sized bowl. Make sure that you remove any pits and squeeze the sections. You should have around ¼ cup of tangerine juice.

Set sections aside. Take a large bowl and add lemon juice, tangerine juice, and olive oil. Mix them and add salt and pepper for flavor, if you prefer.

2. Use paper towels to pat the cress dry. Add watercress, tomatoes, and olives to the bowl containing the tangerine sections (not to be confused with the bowl containing tangerine juice). Toss them lightly.

3. Pour the tangerine juice mixture on top. Mix well and serve.

Prosciutto and Figs Salad

Prep Time: 10 min

Cook Time: 0 min

Serve: 4

Ingredients:

- One 10-12-oz. package fresh baby spinach

- 1 small hot red chili pepper, finely diced

- 1 carton figs, stems removed and quartered

- ½ cup walnuts, coarsely chopped

- 1 tbsp. fresh orange juice

- 1 tbsp. honey

- 4 slices prosciutto, cut into strips

- Shaved parmesan cheese for garnish

Preparation:

1. Take your spinach and divide them into 4 equal portions. Each portion should be on a separate plate and will act as a base. Add quartered prosciutto, figs, and walnuts on each spinach as toppings.

2. For the dressing, take a small bowl and add honey, orange juice, and diced pepper. Add the mixture over the salad.

3. Finally, toss the salad lightly and use parmesan cheese for the garnish.

Garden Vegetables and Chickpeas Salad

Prep Time: 10 min

Cook Time: 0 min

Serve: 4

Ingredients:

- 2 tbsp. freshly squeezed lemon juice

- 1/8 tsp. freshly ground pepper

- 1 cup cubed part-skim mozzarella cheese

- 1 tbsp. fresh basil leaf, snipped

- 1 (15-oz.) can chickpeas, rinsed and well drained

- 2 cups coarsely chopped fresh broccoli

- 2 cloves fresh garlic, finely minced

- ½ cup sliced fresh carrots

- 1 7½-oz. can diced tomatoes, undrained

Preparation:

1. Use a large bowl and add garlic, basil, lemon juice, and ground pepper. Mix them well.

2. Add the chickpeas, carrots, tomatoes with juice, broccoli, and mozzarella cheese. Toos all the ingredients well.

3. You can serve immediately, or you can keep it refrigerated overnight.

Peppered Watercress Salad

Prep Time: 5 min

Cook Time: 0 min

Serve: 4

Ingredients:

- 2 tsp. champagne vinegar

- 2 bunches (about 8 cups) watercress, rinsed and rough stems removed

- 2 tbsp. extra-virgin olive oil

- Salt and freshly ground pepper to taste

Preparation:

1. Drain the watercress properly.

2. Take out a small bowl and then add salt, pepper, vinegar, and olive oil. Mix them well together. Transfer the watercress to a bowl. Add the vinegar mixture into it and toss well. Serve immediately.

Baked egg with cheddar and beef

Prep Time: 20 min

Cook Time: 20 min

Serve: 6

Ingredients:

- Six eggs 1 lb beef

- One chopped green pepper

- Salt to taste

- Pepper to taste

- 1 cup green beans

- Cream of mushroom soup

- 1/2 cup shredded cheddar cheese

- 1 cup almond milk

- 1 tbsp vegetable oil

- 1 cup mushrooms

- 1 tsp onion powder

- 2 tbsp cornstarch

- 1/2 tsp salt

Preparation:

1. Cook beef with beans and bell pepper. Crack eggs and cook for five minutes.

2. Transfer the beef to the casserole and pour mushroom soup and toss. Bake in a preheated oven at 350 degrees for 20 minutes.

Cream of Mushroom Soup:

1. Blend all the items of mushroom soup in the blender.

2. Boil the mixture and simmer it for 12 minutes.

Heavenly egg bake with pancakes

Prep Time: 15 min

Cook Time: 25 min

Serve: 8

Ingredients:

- 2 cups baking mix

- 2 cups shredded Cheddar cheese

- 1 cup milk

- 5 tbsp maple syrup

- Two eggs

- 1.5 tbsp white sugar

- 12 slices cooked bacon

Preparation:

1. Mix all the ingredients in a bowl and bake in a preheated oven at 350 degrees for 25 minutes.

2. Top with cheese and bacon and bake for five more minutes.

Blueberry and vanilla scones

Prep Time: 15 min

Cook Time: 10 min

Serve: 8

Ingredients:

- 1/2 tsp baking powder

- 225 g Self-rising flour

- One pinch of salt

- 2 tbsp soured cream

- One egg

- 50 g caster sugar

- 75 g butter

- 75 g blueberries

- 1 tsp vanilla extract

Preparation:

1. Mix flour, salt, baking powder, sugar, butter, and blueberries in a bowl.

2. Whisk vanilla with cream and egg and add in flour mixture. Make small rounded shapes and bake in a preheated oven at 200 degrees for 15 minutes.

3. Mix strawberries, sugar, and vanilla and make syrup.

4. Pour syrup over baked cookies and serve.

Frittata with brie and bacon

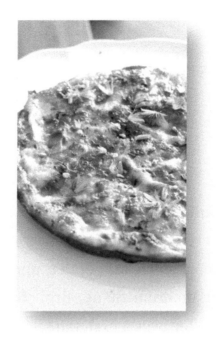

Prep Time: 5 min

Cook Time: 20 min

Serve: 6

Ingredients:

- 1/2 tsp salt

- 1/2 tsp pepper

- 1/2 cup whipping cream

- Eight slices bacon

- Eight eggs

- Two cloves garlic

- 4 oz brie

Preparation:

1. Heat oil in a skillet over medium flame and saute bacon for five minutes. Transfer bacon to plate.

2. Mix egg, cream salt, bacon, pepper, and garlic and cook in heated oil over medium flame. Broil bacon mixture for five minutes in broiler over a high flame.

Coffee with butter

Prep Time: 5 min

Cook Time: 5 min

Serve: 1

Ingredients:

- 1 cup hot coffee
- 2 tbsp butter
- 1 tbsp coconut oil

Preparation:

Combine all the items in a blender and serve.

Lightning Source UK Ltd.
Milton Keynes UK
UKHW020651160421
382097UK00012B/747